SYSTEMA HEALTH

25 PRACTISES
FOR A LIFETIME OF HEALTH, FITNESS AND WELLBEING

First Published in Great Britain 2016 by Mirador Publishing

First edition: 2016

A copy of this work is available through the British Library.

ISBN : 978-1-911473-26-8

Mirador Publishing
10 Greenbrook Terrace
Taunton
Somerset
TA1 1UT

SYSTEMA HEALTH

25 PRACTISES
FOR A LIFETIME OF HEALTH, FITNESS AND WELLBEING

MATT HILL

Warning

CONTENTS

ABOUT THE AUTHOR

Matt Hill is the owner and chief instructor at his Systema School in Wiltshire, UK. He started training in the Martial Arts in 1987 and by 1991 he was living as a full time student of Aikido giant Morihiro Saito in Iwama, Japan, where he lived for two years. Matt began his study of Systema in 2003. Matt is a qualified Systema Instructor under Vladimir Vasiliev, a 5th degree black belt in Aikido and an ex-Parachute Regiment Captain. He teaches full time at his school as well as leading workshops throughout the UK, Europe and the Middle East. He is committed to his personal training and sharing the gift of Systema with as many people as possible.

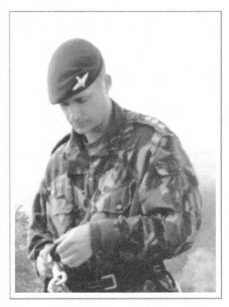

For more information, complimentary newsletters, details on seminars, training camps and instructional materials, visit
www.matthill.co.uk

ACKNOWLEDGEMENTS

They say that progression in anything is 1% inspiration and 99% perspiration. Actually, I have found that it is by the perspiration and support of many others, that real progress is achieved.

There are several people without whom this book would not have started. Mikhail Ryabko and Vladimir Vasiliev. I can't thank them enough for their guidance, example, genius and the willingness to share that with the world. Their experience and skill is hard won and they share it so openly and generously.

My special thanks also go to Haden Scott, Jason Rodwell, Karl Durrant, Gareth Leake and Kim Seviour for their help with the book. Specific thanks to Daniel Satari for his patience, skill and craftsmanship in helping to bring this book to life.

I could not pass this opportunity without thanking the Saito family in Iwama, Japan for kindling my passion for the Martial Arts and giving me so much at a very young age that has stayed with me. I would also like to thank my parents, for their continued love and support.

I also wish to thank my students, for allowing me to share with them my love and passion for Systema.

Lastly I would like to thank my wife Sarah, for her ongoing support and gentle encouragement to actually get this book finished to a deadline! Without her, it would still be sitting in a 'To Do' list.

FOREWORD BY VLADIMIR VASILIEV

DIRECTOR AND CHIEF INSTRUCTOR OF SYSTEMA HEADQUARTERS, TORONTO, CANADA

I would like to congratulate Matt on this publication.

It is always good to have an experienced professional become a Systema instructor.

In the time that I have known Matt, he has proved himself a strong and caring person, and a talented instructor.

Matt has been closely following the training methods taught by Mikhail Ryabko and myself. His understanding, willingness, and ability to share are very impressive.

Systema practice is beneficial for people of all ages and capabilities and Matt exemplifies this well in his teaching and in this publication.

Systema is now a widespread art, taught all over the world. I hope that with Matt's book more people will strengthen their health and martial art skills.

Vladimir Vasiliev, Toronto.
24th June 2016.

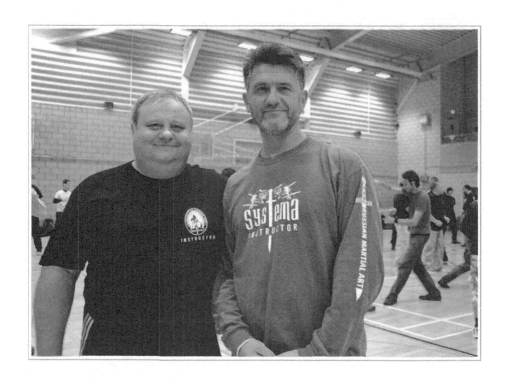

Systema Founder Mikhail Ryabko (left) and Systema HQ Director Vladimir Vasiliev in 2014 at the 'Legends of Systema' Seminar in Shropshire, in the United Kingdom. Mikhail and Vladimir are the two men largely responsible for the spread and popularity of Systema around the world.

INTRODUCTION

Simple tools for a lifetime of health and wellbeing

The roots of Systema go back ten centuries to the warriors and monasteries of Orthodox ancient Russia. Systema began to grow in popularity around the time of the collapse of the Soviet Union. Its popularity in recent times is largely due to two men: Mikhail Ryabko and Vladimir Vasiliev. Mikhail is a highly decorated Russian Army Colonel who received training from the age of five. From the age of fifteen he received combative training. He has been in numerous military campaigns and holds many medals and awards. He is the Master Teacher of Systema. Born in Russia Vladimir Vasiliev received intensive combative training and profound Systema training from Mikhail Ryabko. Vladimir is an exceptional student of Mikhail, and a decorated combat veteran. Since 1993 Vladimir has been based in Toronto, Canada and has been largely responsible for Systema's rapid growth outside Russia. Vladimir has trained and certified well over 600 instructors and schools in over 40 countries.

Systema or, 'The System', is a complete approach to health, wellbeing and self-defence. It deals with the physical, psychological or emotional and spiritual aspects of your wellbeing. It is a holistic method of improving your life. "How can a system be both I hear you ask?" Well, as Vladimir Vasiliev puts it, a good warrior is a healthy warrior, in body, mind and spirit for the whole of his life.

To really benefit from all that Systema has to offer, it should become a way of living, or being. You have to have faith in sacrificing old ways and habits of breathing, moving and thinking. Training is not solely limited to classes. It will naturally spill out into everyday life. Be hungry of spirit and willing to discover new skills, feelings and horizons within yourself. It's a journey and not a destination and each step on the journey is filled with unexpected benefits. Many people describe Systema as a cleaning system. A way to remove your mind, body and spirit of the tension, fears and anxieties that daily living puts in. Tension restricts your movement, thought, action and sense of ease and peace and when that tension becomes chronic, your very life expectancy also becomes limited.

I feel very much like a beginner on this journey. Every day I enquire deeper into myself through Systema. In the pages of this book, I have outlined some of the health enhancing practises that I have learned from my teachers. I hope that it will support beginners who are just starting their Systema journey and beginners like myself, who have been studying for much longer. It is my hope, that readers will use these practises to enquire deeper of themselves and as a guide to share Systema with others.

It is important to note that this book is not meant to replace a teacher. Even if you do not have a teacher locally enough to train regularly you should try to get to seminars with a recognized Systema Instructor. Development in Systema requires guidance and support, from someone with a deep knowledge and understanding of its methods and principles. How do I find that person? Thats easy. Take a look at their students.

Lastly, I would say this. Training in Systema is fun. It brings deep joy and a sense of peace. Enquire deeply, train with every fibre of your being. Try to live it, in every movement and breath and your progress and health will surely improve. As Vladimir Vasiliev says, "The beauty of Systema, is that as your skill improves, so does your health."

I have created a video for each of the practises that is free for owners of the book. You can view the videos by using this link: http://www.matthill.co.uk/systema-health

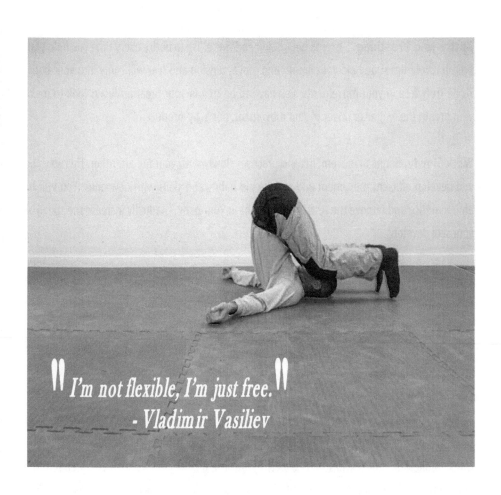

I'm not flexible, I'm just free.
- Vladimir Vasiliev

TRAINING TOOLS

A compass and map for your journey

Notice your breathing. Systema begins and ends here. Try to notice every time you hold your breath. Every time you hold your breath and move, tension and fear will come into your body. To be truly free in your movements, you have to be free in your breath. Always look to make your breath the engine or driver of your movement, not a 'by-product' of it.

Work Slowly. Begin all movements and practises slowly with your full attention. This way you will develop efficient movement and replace old habits and skills with new ones. You will be able to notice and remove the restrictive tensions in your body. Gradually increase the speed as your skill develops.

Adjust the volume. As your skill develops, you will want to go faster. This is fine. Notice when you get stuck. Maybe your breathing stops, your movements seizes up, you run out of ideas, you repeat patterns over and over again, or any other aspect that causes frustration. At these times slow down again. Build and wire new skill and understanding and then gradually speed up again.

Strive for creativity in your training. Remember that Systema is not training for a set sequence of movements, such as a Kata or gymnastics competition. This is a much more transferable skill, that reaches every aspect of life. The pictures in this book are intended as a guide only and just show one way of doing things. Play and experiment. If you can do it forwards, try it backwards, or with your eyes closed, or on a balance beam etc. Have fun but stay safe. My deep desire, is that through the logical progressions in these practises, you will begin freely creating your own practises, to the extent where you are training in Systema in every moment. By all means use my progressions as a guide, but you then have to just move randomly and naturally. Try not to form patterns in your movements.

Movement. Systema is really the study of movement. Freedom and ease of movement is your aim. As your movement relaxes, so will your psyche. Then your health will improve exponentially.

Search for the struggle. You will inevitably find sticky points in your movement. Ranges of motion that you can't move through without momentum, if at all. Areas where you hold your breath through strain and tension. S*earch for these areas and spend time in them.* You will iron them out much faster this way.

A film is worth a million words. Video yourself doing the movements. You will correct yourself so much faster when you can see your movement yourself. Vladimir Vasiliev offers a video coaching program through his website that is well worth using.

Do the pillars once every day (Practices 11-14). If I could give you one tip for a healthy body and movement for the rest of your life, it would be this one. Do the pillars once a day. One of each pillar. Once. As slow as you can, with full range of motion, working on breathing and relaxing your body. The whole of Systema is in these movements.

Look for Symmetry. Look to get as good on your left side as your right side in all the practices. Don't favour one side over another.

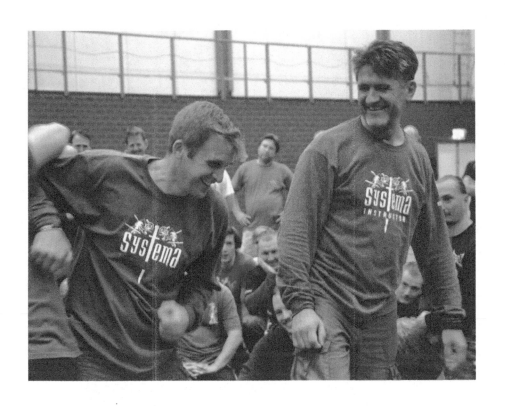

Training in Systema is fun, it brings deep joy and a sense of peace.

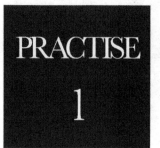
PRACTISE 1

SYSTEMA HEALTH PRACTISES
BREATH WORK

"God shaped man from the soil of the ground and blew the breath of life into his nostrils, and man became a living being" Genesis 2:7

Breathwork is the first thing that I will cover in this book. Systema begins with breathwork. Therefore our first practise, is the first skill. In life, the very first thing that we do is inhale and the last thing that we do is exhale. Every moment in between, involves breathing. A better understanding of your breathing, and practice in mastering it, can create dramatic changes in the quality of your life.

There are three phases of breath. Inhale, exhale and hold. We will deal with all three in this section. In Systema there are three basic things to remember when it comes to breathing.

- ❖ *Inhale through the nose.*
- ❖ *Exhale through the mouth (when under physical or mental stress or strain) and;*
- ❖ *Don't stop or hold your breath.*

You will be amazed when you notice just how often you hold your breath. You will probably hold your breath when doing something even mildly strenuous, like sitting down or standing up. When thinking or concentrating, or when taken by an emotion such as fear or surprise. The key aim of correct breathing is to calm and relax you. There are also some real health benefits to breathing correctly through the nose, as opposed to the mouth:

- ❖ *It filters the air catching dirt and dust particles on the nasal hairs and mucus membrane.*
- ❖ *It activates your immune system.*
- ❖ *It cools and optimises the pituitary gland, one of the main hormone production centres in the body.*
- ❖ *It warms the air to 35 degrees centigrade, the optimum temperature for the air to be absorbed through the lung wall and into the blood stream.*

- ❖ *It stimulates the body's production of Nitric Oxide (NO) gas, which is a natural relaxant and a cousin of laughing gas.*
- ❖ *It helps to keep the sinus passage clear to keep the brain cool and avoid sinus problems.*
- ❖ *It aids early detection of harmful substances*
- ❖ *It aids intuition and decision-making, we can smell fear and danger.*

❖ *It interrupts the panic cycle. When our thoughts start to escalate and spin out of control in times of high stress or danger, an inhale through the nose interrupts this and allows you to bring your breathing and thoughts back under control.*

Finally and crucially, it activates the para-sympathetic nervous system, your rest and digest state. This is opposed to the sympathetic nervous system, your fight or flight state. By activating the para-sympathetic nervous system, we do several crucial things. We:

❖ *Lower the heart rate.*

❖ *Lower the blood pressure.*

❖ *Relax the muscles.*

❖ *Allow for calmer, clearer thinking.*

❖ *Open up our senses (sight, sound) avoiding tunnel vision and the 'rushing or pounding' sound of blood in the ears.*

❖ *Normalise our perception of time, space and reason.*

We will cover three breath cycles to help you induce calm into your system: *Circular breath, triangular breath and square breath.*

BREATH PRACTISE: CIRCULAR BREATH

In the circular breath, we inhale then we exhale. A continuous circle.

Note that under non-stressful circumstances, it is fine and good to inhale and exhale through the nose.

As a basic rule the longer, smoother and quieter the inhale and exhale, the more relaxed you will become. Try to aim for inhaling for six-seconds and exhaling for six-seconds. This is five breaths per minute and a good baseline for relaxation. Begin by lying on the floor. This is the most relaxed position to start. There will be minimum muscular tension. It also leaves the system with the minimum work to do in terms of pushing blood around the body. The fluids in the body will level and balance. It is the most restful position. Begin inhaling through the nose and out through the mouth.

The aim on the inhale, is to minimise the amount of tension that comes into the body. Try to inhale straight into the bottom of the lungs. This will inflate the stomach (see FIG. 1 below) rather than the chest as the diaphragm moves down. This is called diaphragmatic breathing. It is the type of breathing used by singers and martial artists among others, to relax and provide steadiness and power. Especially, try to keep the shoulders, chest and back relaxed as you inhale.

As you exhale, the stomach falls (see FIG. 1 below). Allow gravity to push the air out. Try to completely relax your muscles and your system. Physically, mentally and emotionally you 'clean' yourself of tension and stress.

Fig. 1: Inhale

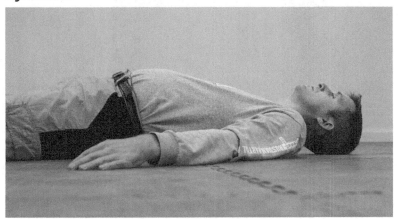

Fig. 2: Exhale

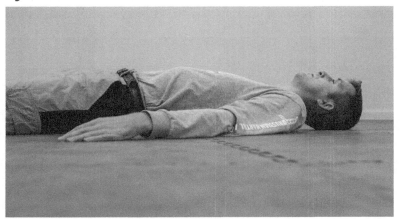

IMPORTANT: *The volume of air should be the same on each count of the breath. So it is smooth and even across the length, not a big gulp at the start and then slowing toward the end.*

Notice in the picture, that there is not even tension around the mouth, to release the air out on the exhale. You simply allow the air to escape from the lips. Think of the mouth like a 'one-way' valve. As you inhale though the nose the mouth is closed, as you exhale through the mouth this opens the mouth. As soon as your exhale completes this naturally closes the mouth again. There are no big or tense 'blowing' movements.

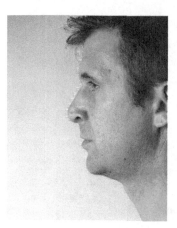 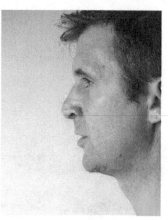

INHALE CALM   **EXHALE TENSION**

TRIANGULAR BREATH

I mentioned at the start there are three phases to the breath. An inhale, an exhale and a hold. In the triangular breath we introduce the hold. Earlier I wrote that we never hold the breath in Systema. There is one exception to this rule. We hold it when it serves a purpose. This will be covered more in the next practice: *holds and recovery*.

In the triangular hold we do an inhale followed by a hold then an exhale. Try to progress to comfortably reach a six-second inhale, followed by a six-second hold, then a six-second exhale.

IMPORTANT: Don't 'snatch' the breath when you inhale after the hold. The inhale should be smooth.

Do a few minutes of this and then follow it with an empty hold, i.e. INHALE – EXHALE – HOLD. This will add slightly more stress to the system, as you are now holding the breath after an exhalation. In the beginning, it may be difficult to do long smooth breaths, as many people are used to short, shallow breaths. Persevere and very quickly, you will begin to be able to extend the length of your breaths to a count of 6, 10, 15 or more seconds per phase.

SQUARE BREATH
The last of the breath cycles is a square breath. INHALE – HOLD – EXHALE – HOLD. This is actually the normal breathing pattern for most people: an inhale, followed by a short hold, then an exhale, followed by a short hold. Try to do a pattern of 2 seconds per phase, then 3 and then 4 etc. Try to get up to 10 seconds or more per phase. If you can do 15 seconds per phase, you are up to one complete breath per minute. Use the holds to find relaxation in yourself, use subtle movement in the body to identify the tension and then release it during the phases.

To view the free video of this practise please use the link below:
http://www.matthill.co.uk/systema-health

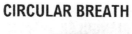

CIRCULAR BREATH

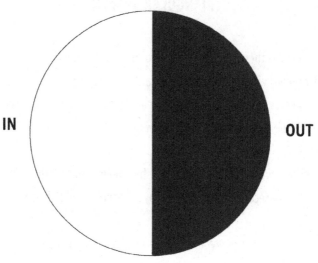

IN   OUT

TRIANGULAR BREATH

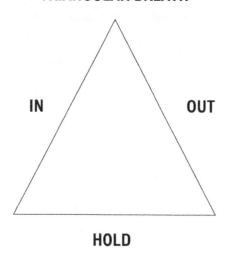

IN   OUT

HOLD

SQUARE BREATH

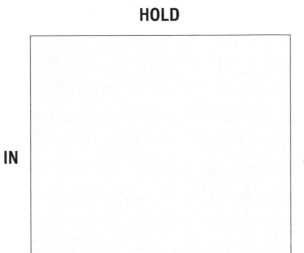

HOLD

IN ___ **OUT**

HOLD

Note: I have used six second phases in most instances to illustrate the cycles. This is a benchmark and for most people will provide a good balance for being relaxed and aware. It is important however, to experiment with longer and shorter cycles as appropriate for you.

PRACTISE 2

BREATH HOLDS AND RECOVERY

Increasing your bandwidth for dealing with stress, anxiety & fear

Breath holds and recovery are very simple and reliable ways to understand how to restore yourself. The breath hold is a method of introducing stress to your system. The longer the hold, the more the stress. Very quickly, you will begin to feel an increasing level of panic through the breath hold. This panic will be emotional and physical. Your goal is to stay calm, relaxed and through movement, release the tension as it builds in your body. You will feel the panic 'clutch' at your body, making it convulse or tense in areas. Try to move these areas or soften them out, so that the panic recedes. The feeling of panic comes in waves. If you can get over the first one (this is the hardest), then the next ones are slightly easier.

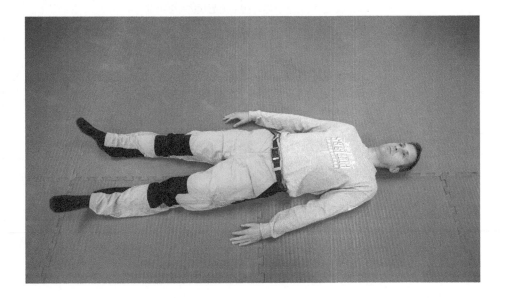

Begin the exercise lying down. Do some normal breath cycles (circle, triangle and square) to relax yourself. The hold can be done on four stages of the breath.

1. A full inhale – take in a full breath.
2. A soft inhale – just take in a normal breath.
3. A soft exhale – just do a normal out breath.
4. A full exhale – take a full out breath.

THE RECOVERY. The most important part of the hold is the recovery. Here you need to do 'burst breathing'. This is a short inhale through the nose, followed by a short exhale through the mouth. This is repeated until your biorhythms (heart rate, blood pressure, emotional state,

31

tensions, etc.) start to return to normal. You then gradually lengthen and smooth out the breath. The breathing starts fast, like a dog panting or a woman in labour. It is important that straight after the hold, the first breath is not a big gulp. You should go straight into 'burst breathing' (a repeated short inhale followed by a short exhale). In periods of intense stress, such as combat, pain, shock or trauma, a recovery or 'burst' breath, literally gives you the breath by breath capability to continue to function. Short sips of air are the best way to recover in this instance.

To view the free video of this practise please use the link below:
http://www.matthill.co.uk/systema-health

"The beauty of Systema is that it provides you with health and skill at the same time."

- Vladimir Vasiliev

PRACTISE 3

BREATH LADDERS

Our natural 'reset' button

Breath ladders are a great way to practise walking and running, with minimal tension and with deep calming breaths. You learn to 'clean' yourself of tension as you move, so that your walk is stable and solid; neither floppy nor tense. As with the prone breath cycles, you can do any breath pattern. A good start point is to try to go from 1 up to 10 and then back down to 1. So you inhale for one step, then exhale for 1 step. Then you inhale for 2 steps, exhale for 2 steps. Inhale for 3, exhale for 3. All the way up to 10 steps inhale and 10 steps exhale. Then you come back down 9, 8, 7 etc. all the way to 1. When you have completed this forwards, then try it backwards. You can also try it with the breath cycles shown in practise 1. Combining your breathing and your walking is a critical stage to master early in Systema. It shows you how to recover yourself from stress and trauma and it also shows you how to keep movement in your body to aid recovery. When the stress level is high, you should focus on one step inhale, one step exhale, gradually lengthening and smoothing out, as you calm the body, mind and emotions. As you walk, subtly check your body for tension with movement of the shoulders, arms, hips, legs etc. Check that your muscles are not tight by wobbling them. If you can feel them wobble, it is a good indication that they are relaxed.

During the running stage, try to run in a way that relaxes all of your muscles. Vladimir Vasiliev states that there are traditionally only two reasons to run. Out of fear, and to relax. This is a run to show you how to relax. The arms are loose (imagine them as ropes tied to your shoulders with a heavy knot in the end. They should jangle as you run). Then try to get this feeling of looseness in the muscles into your whole body. You should be able to bring your attention to all muscles and joints in the body and feel them wobbling around as you run. Do the same breathing patterns with the running, as you did with the walking including going backwards.

IMPORTANT: It is important that you practice going backwards. When you first try this, you will be apprehensive about walking into something or falling over. Practise relaxing (especially the shoulders and hips) and try not to look over your shoulder. Go slowly, in a safe place and learn to relax. In a combat situation, you will probably spend as much time going backwards as forwards. Endeavour to get comfortable moving in a smooth relaxed manner in every way that you can.

Walking is a great 'reset button' for the body. Much like turning a computer off and then back on again when it freezes. Linking your walking with your breathing and focusing on relaxation, can be used to calm and restore your body, mind and spirit in times of need.

To view the free video of this practise please use the link below:
http://www.matthill.co.uk/systema-health

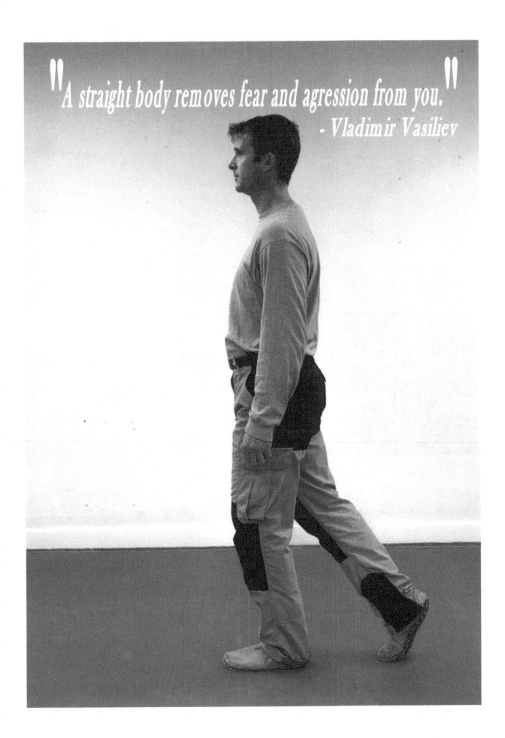

"*A straight body removes fear and agression from you.*"
- Vladimir Vasiliev

PRACTISE 4

GROUND MOVEMENT

Build your body from the ground up

In Systema we build a body from the ground up, just as you did when you were a baby. You explored your body, movement and surroundings from the horizontal position. First on your back, then on your front. The best way to get soft, free movement back into your body at any age, is to begin in these positions again.

We begin on the back. The key aim with these movements is to soften the muscles and the connections between the muscles. One way to do this is by 'reaching' rather than 'pushing' into movements.

Exercise

Begin by extending the heels away from the body. Try not to tense the muscles, just soften, relax and let them slide as they extend. Do this on an exhale. Then inhale as you come back to a neutral starting position. Do this several times. Then do the same with the head. Again try it several times.

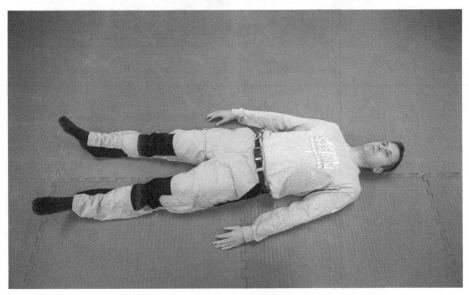

RELAXED TO START

Then try it with both the heels and the head at the same time.

HEELS OUT   **HEAD OUT**

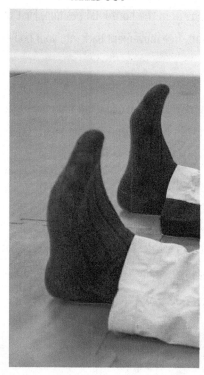 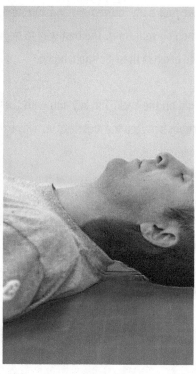

Then begin to reach with the hands and feet. In the beginning keep the right leg and right arm on the right side of the body and the left arm and left leg on the left side of the body. Reach one limb at a time. Allow the movement to pull not just the limb but where it attaches to the body. So for example, as you reach with the right arm, allow it to release and pull the shoulder, neck, back, side and even your hip and leg. Gradually progress to moving two or more limbs at a time.

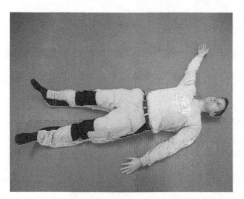 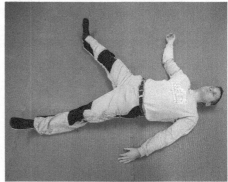

Progression. Then begin reaching across the body with the limbs. For example, bring the right arm across the chest to the left gradually pulling the body off the floor as the arm reaches. Explore your freedom of movement in all ranges and angles. Try to exhale as you reach and inhale as you return to neutral and vice versa.

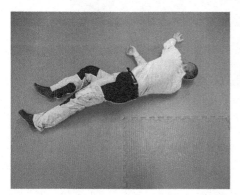 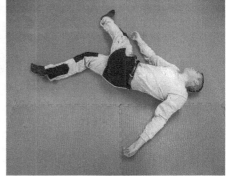

Important. *It is imperative that you begin to get freedom and creativity in your movement. By all means use my progressions as a guide, but you then have to just move randomly and naturally. Try not to form patterns in your movements.*

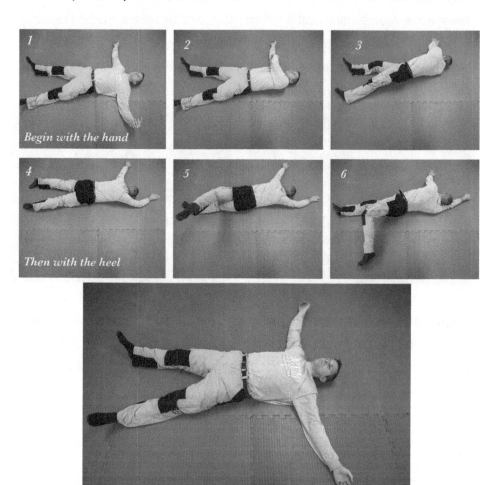

Next try to do a 'sausage roll'. Try to do this with the least amount of effort possible. Imagine that you are unconscious. That you are being pulled by your hand from your back onto your front. Your body should be heavy and relaxed. Your hand moves first as it is pulled, followed by your forearm, then upper arm, then shoulder, then back, hip, leg and finally, once your body reaches a 'tipping point', you will flop over. As you return, use the same arm in the opposite direction. Again begin with the hand and try to get the sequential engagement of each muscle in the movement. Then try the other side. Then try it with the feet.

Do this very slowly, super slowly. Get the sensitivity to tension in your body. Over time you can gradually increase the speed. Only go as fast as you can move, before tension comes into your movement. When you find this speed, ease back ever so slightly until there is no tension and smooth it out. Then increase the speed again when you feel comfortable.

To view the free video of this practise please use the link below:
http://www.matthill.co.uk/systema-health

PRACTISE

5

ROPE TWISTS

A great practice to find tension in the body

It is very important to go slowly. If you go fast you will miss the benefits. It is only by going slow that you will find your tension, soften the muscles and remove it.

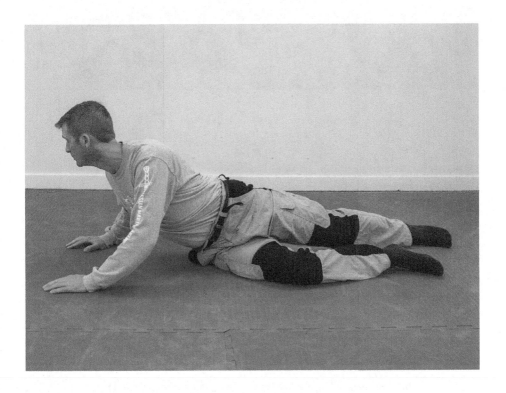

Important:

Exhale before you start moving. Let the breath lead the movement and move inside your breath. This way you soften and protect your body from tension and strain.

It is also important to make sure that you do the two movements of turning and going from sitting to prone at the same time.

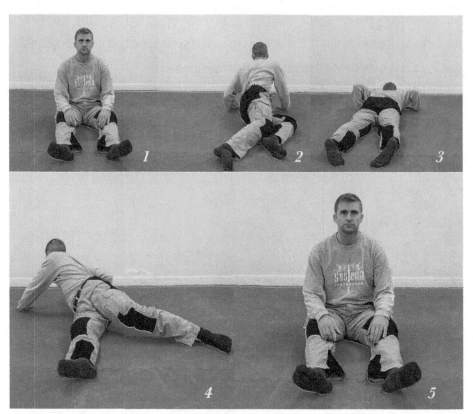

Begin sitting on the floor with your legs out straight in front of you. You are going to turn around and lie down on your front in the prone position. You will lead the movement with your eyes. Start to turn the head by looking behind you. Try to move the head and neck as far as they will go, before you start moving the shoulders. Then do the same with the shoulders before the back starts to move. Follow this principle through the body from head, shoulders, back, hip, thigh and knee to foot. This will teach the skill of moving the body sequentially.

To return to sitting, lead the movement with the heel. Reach across your body with the heel until it starts to pull your knee, thigh, hip, back, shoulder and head, bringing you back to the sitting position. This movement twists the whole body and this will find tension, allowing you to soften it out with your breath.

' LEAD WITH THE BREATH '

To view the free video of this practise please use the link below:
http://www.matthill.co.uk/systema-health

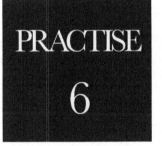

PRACTISE 6

FREE GROUND MOVEMENT

Combining practises

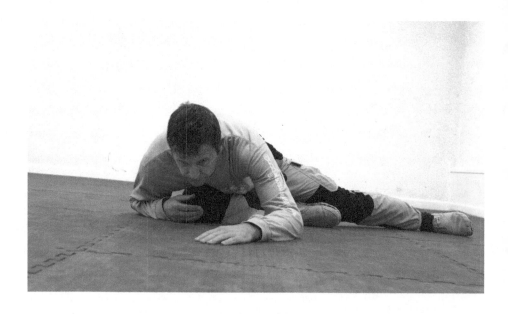

Now combine the ground movement, sausage rolls and rope twists practises all together in free movement. Inhale for one movement and exhale for one movement. This is your chance to be creative and free in your ground movement. Go slowly and find the sticky points in terms of tension. Look for where your breath catches and the ranges of movement where you lose control of your body. Go slowly through these areas and iron them out. *Search for the struggle and spend time there.*

As with all of the practises, as you improve this ability to move freely on the ground you can gradually speed up. Beware of tension. As soon as you get tense, ease back and smooth yourself out again. Being smooth is more important than being fast here.

Rolls are great for self confidence and self massage of the muscles, especially around the shoulders and back; areas that are hard to reach by yourself.

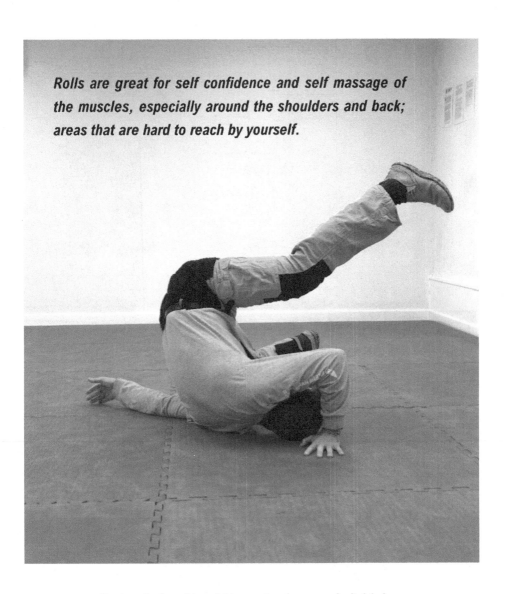

To view the free video of this practise please use the link below:

http://www.matthill.co.uk/systema-health

PRACTISE 7

SUPERMAN TO TORTOISE

Advanced practise

This is a good exercise to test your core movement and tension under strain. It is more advanced than the sausage roll, due to the extra strain on the body.

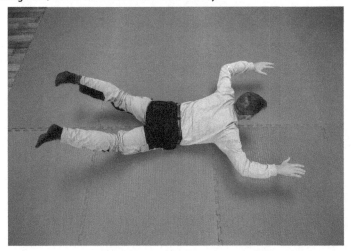

Begin on your tummy and slowly raise your arms and legs off the ground until only the abdomen is in contact. Then rotate until only the bum is on the floor. Then return to the tummy. As always, it is important to lead with an exhalation and to find and remove tension from the movement. Symmetry is important so make sure that you rotate to both left and right.

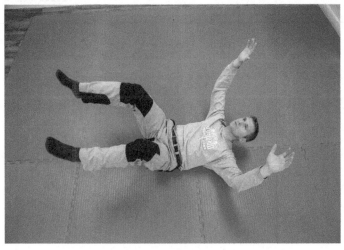

To view the free video of this practise please use the link below:
http://www.matthill.co.uk/systema-health

*"Tension in your body
is a manifestation of
fear at some level."*
- *Mikhail Ryabko*

PRACTISE 8

KNEES BACK KNEES

Learning to fall softly

Begin in a kneeling position.

Exhale and then start to drop the body into a foetal position and roll onto your side. This should be under control and only the soft parts (muscles not bones) of your body should contact the floor. Then extend yourself out fully onto your back.

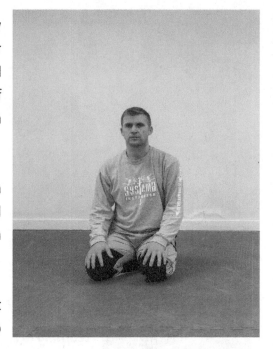

At this point inhale through the nose, then continue the movement back to a foetal position the other side and then to a kneeling position again.

A nice side effect, is that this movement will teach you to fall softly and roll to avoid injury to the body.

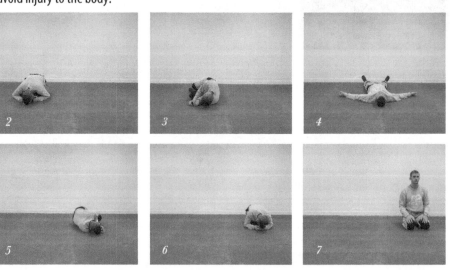

To view the free video of this practise please use the link below:
http://www.matthill.co.uk/systema-health

"Progress comes in hills and plateaus. Understand this and your approach to Training becomes much more relaxed."
- Matt Hill

PRACTISE

9

BUM SHUFFLE

A fun core exercise

Sit on your bum with hands and feet off the floor (FIG 1). Then, walk on your bum without making contact with the ground with any other part of the body. Try walking forwards and then backwards.

When you can do this, then try to move sideways. Try to do this with a jump or hop (FIG 2). Move to the left and to the right and then also try the diagonals. You should be able to move along all the main compass angles from a central point. As always remember to breathe and relax as much as possible. This works your core stability, relaxation, balance and strength.

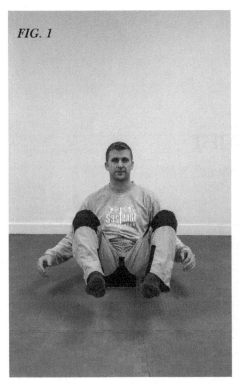
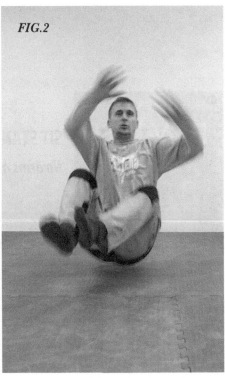

FIG. 1

FIG.2

To view the free video of this practise please use the link below:
http://www.matthill.co.uk/systema-health

PRACTISE 10

SIT STAND TEST

No arms allowed!

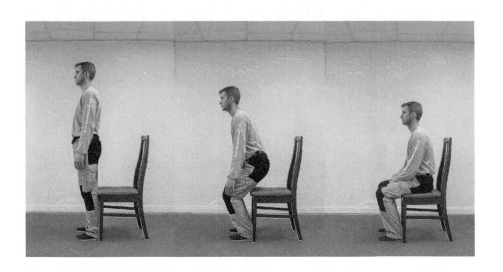

This test used to be used by doctors as a simple way to check strength to body weight ratio, motor coordination, tension levels, balance and blood pressure for people in their 70's.

Very simply people had to lower themselves under control onto a chair and then stand up again, in balance and without feeling dizzy. You are not allowed to use your arms for support at all in the movement.

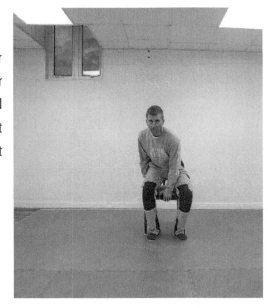

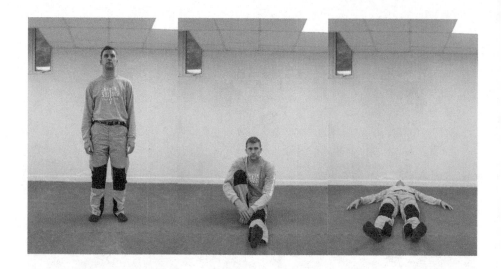

For people of a younger age the test is a little more difficult. The Challenge is to sit on the floor and then stand up again without using your knees, hands or elbows. So the only contact is with the feet, backs of legs and the bum. Challenge! You start with 10 points and every time you have to use another body part, or the movement is not under control or balanced, you lose a point. Studies show that the closer you get to a full 10 points, the better your longevity!

In the pictures, I am seen going down with one leg bent and the other straight in a pistol (of course you can do it cross legged if you wish) and going into a prone position, This is slightly harder and by all means try this too.

PLEASE TRY THIS AT HOME

To view the free video of this practise please use the link below:
http://www.matthill.co.uk/systema-health

THE FOUR PILLARS OF HUMAN MOVEMENT

Push up, Sit up, Leg raise, Squat
Search for the struggle

CHECKING FOR FREEDOM IN YOUR MOVEMENT

The four pillars are multi-purpose and are probably the oldest and most enduring of all static physical exercises, and for good reason. You will have been doing these in one form or another since you were a toddler or even younger.

When doing them in Systema, check your body for freedom from tension. To do this see if you can move your body, try small wiggling or wobbling movements, especially the areas under tension. Be sure to breathe freely throughout the whole range of the movement. The four pillars check your strength and smoothness of movement, by seeing if you can complete the full range of movement slowly, under control at the same slow speed for the full range.

For all the pillars, try to do the movement for a count of 20 seconds down and 20 seconds up. So for example, in the push up try to take 10 seconds to bend your arms half way down and a further 10 seconds to touch the floor with your nose, then without rest, take 10 seconds to go back to a 90 degree bend at the elbow and then a further 10 seconds to get to straight arms. So each quarter of the movement takes 10 seconds. It is important to work to be able to go at a constant slow speed at each stage. Don't be tempted to go fast through the hard bits.

You will increase your strength in these exercises and balance out your body on a macro and micro level. On a macro level you will balance your upper body and arms (push up) lower body (squat) core and front of the body (sit up) and core and back of the body (leg raise). On a micro level, you balance strength and stability through the individual muscles during the concentric and eccentric phases of movement.

The real aim is to learn to relax under strain can you move, or are you as stiff as a board? Can you move AND breathe throughout the movement? Go slow. *Search for the struggle.*

If you notice intense shaking of the muscles and trembling this is normal. It can be just muscle fatigue, or a good sign that stress is leaving the body.

Push up

Sit up

Leg raise

Squat

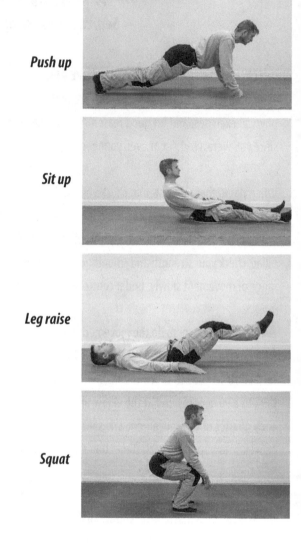

To view the free video of this practise please use the link below:

http://www.matthill.co.uk/systema-health

PRACTISE 11

THE PUSH UP

Begin in the push up position. You will notice a few things different from the common version of a push up. The whole body is relaxed, not tense as in a typical military style push up (see picture). Also, I am on my fists. This is because at its heart, Systema is a martial art and by using the fists you develop the right angles and structure for the fist to support the body under load, as in a punch. It is of course fine to do it on your hands if the fist is too painful, weak, or you are simply doing it for health benefits. Lower the body slowly and smoothly, breathing smoothly throughout, taking 10 seconds to bend the arms to 90 degrees.

Then take a further 10 seconds to touch the floor with the nose. Then without rest, take another 10 seconds to raise the body, until the arms are at 90 degrees again and then a further 10 seconds to straighten the arms. If this is difficult to begin with try 'burst breathing' (see practise 2) throughout the entire movement.

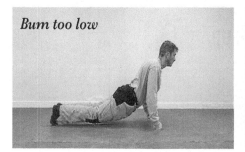
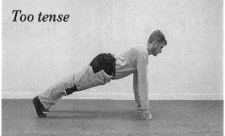

Incorrect positions for the pushup

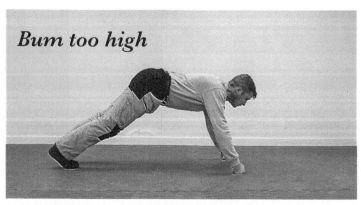

Correct positions for the pushup

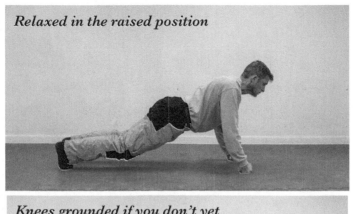

Relaxed in the raised position

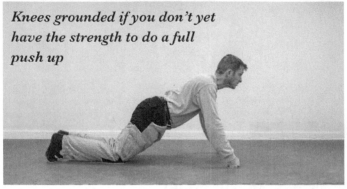

Knees grounded if you don't yet have the strength to do a full push up

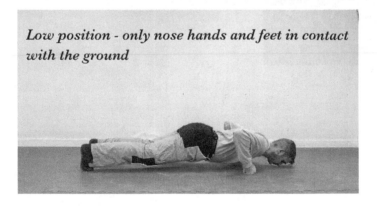

Low position - only nose hands and feet in contact with the ground

If a full push up is too difficult in the beginning, it is fine to do the push up from the knees (as per the middle picture)

To view the free video of this practise please use the link below:

http://www.matthill.co.uk/systema-health

PRACTISE 12

THE SIT UP

In the sit up, you are looking at all of the same things as the push up.

Begin sitting on your bum with legs out in front of you. Proceed to lower yourself backwards, arms relaxed by your side or on your lap and legs on the floor. Legs can have a slight bend at the knee to promote relaxation. Once you have gone all the way down proceed to sit up again keeping the feet on the floor and the arms relaxed.

Once again, try to do the movement slowly and smoothly, breathing throughout the movement to a count of 20 seconds down and 20 seconds up. Ten seconds for each quarter of the movement.

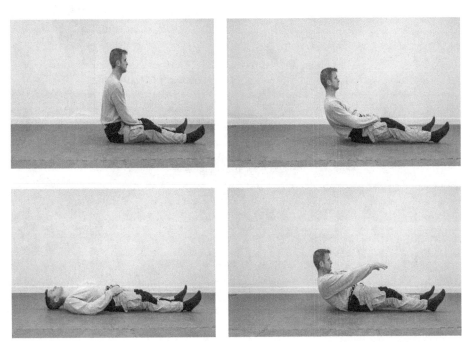

Incorrect position for arms.
Keep arms and legs relaxed throughout the practise.

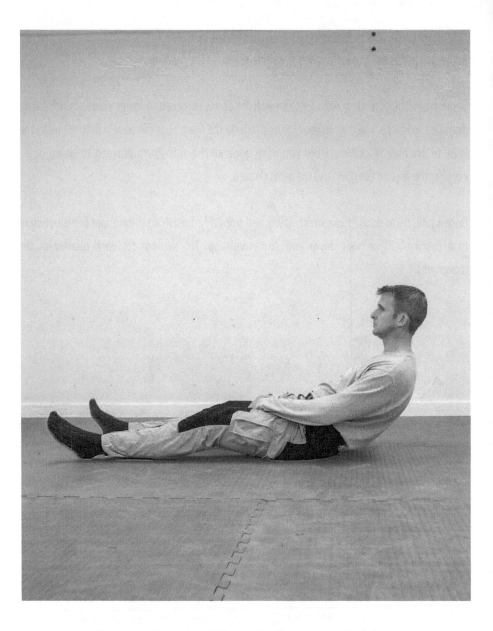

To view the free video of this practise please use the link below:

http://www.matthill.co.uk/systema-health

PRACTISE
13

THE LEG RAISE

In the leg raise, you are again looking at all the same things as the previous pillars. Begin lying down on your back. To protect and support your lower back, you can place your arms palms down under your bum (see FIG 2). Once you progress, you can put your arms by your side or by the side (see FIG 1) of your head. Have a slight bend in the knees.

Fig. 1.

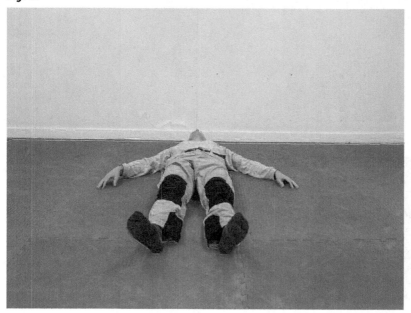

Fig. 2.

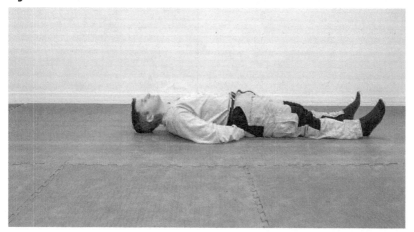

Slowly raise your legs to 90 degrees and then try to keep raising them up and over the head, until they can touch the floor behind the head. Then try to take a deep calming breath whilst you have the legs as far over as you can. Then slowly bring them back over and down to the prone position. Try to move slowly, maintaining the same speed throughout.

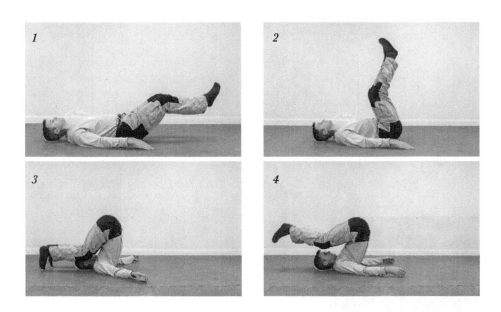

To view the free video of this practise please use the link below:
http://www.matthill.co.uk/systema-health

PRACTISE
14

THE SQUAT

Again, with the squat we are looking at all the same things as the other pillars. Begin in a neutral standing position. Feet should be shoulder width apart and both feet facing forwards. Begin to slowly lower yourself, keeping your back straight and head up (top picture).

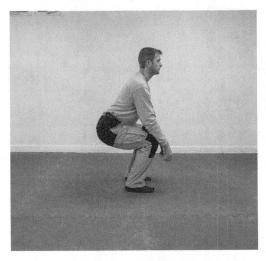

Try not to let the knees go further forwards than the toes. Keep the movement smooth and continuous. Try to keep the legs 'even' as you lower. By this I mean try not to let the knees narrow in towards each other or push out wider than the feet.

Also try to keep the whole of the foot flat on the floor as you move. To do this you will need to relax the legs as much as you can. Too much tension and you will rise onto the balls of the feet, rock back onto the heels, pronate onto the inside edge of the foot, or supinate onto the outside edge of the foot.

Try to squat until your torso rests on your thighs and your arms are on the floor. This is not a question of flexibility or balance, but one of relaxation.

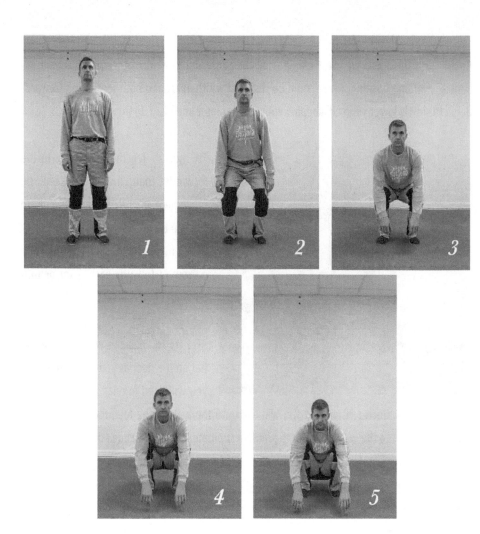

Over time, you should try to get comfortable in this position. It is a natural human position. You will notice that toddlers spend a lot of time in this position and many cultures and countries (especially in the East) still do. It is good for the legs and hips, keeping them balanced and strong through the full range of their motion. It also releases the lower back. Finally, it provides gentle movement and massage for the viscera and helps to squeeze the colon, facilitating colonic evacuation.

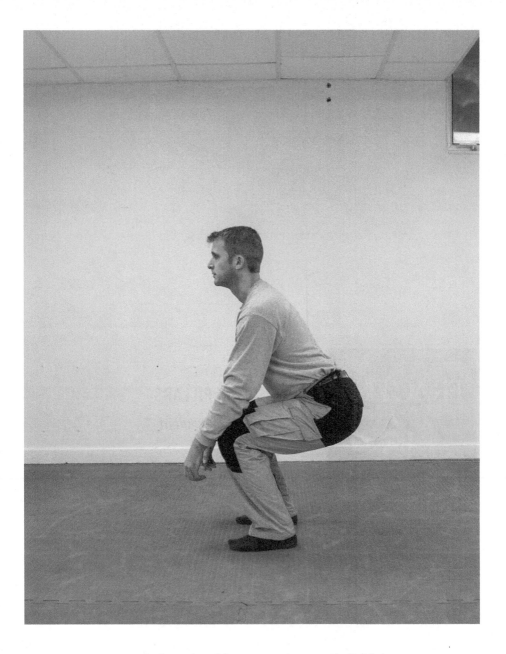

To view the free video of this practise please use the link below:

http://www.matthill.co.uk/systema-health

PRACTISE

15

COMBINATION PILLARS

Free & creative movement

In this practise we combine all four pillars into free, creative movement. Do them in any order and try to vary them, so that you work different ranges of motion through different angles and widths etc.

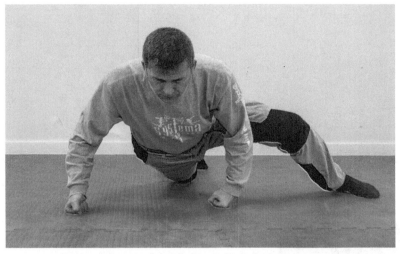

Try to make your breath the engine of your movement,
not a by-product of it.

Focus on your breath for each movement. Inhale on one movement, exhale on the next. This will help with relaxation and endurance.

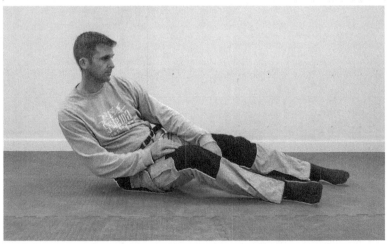

To view the free video of this practise please use the link below:
http://www.matthill.co.uk/systema-health

PRACTISE 16

STRUCTURE STAND AND WALK

This practise focuses on your structure, while standing and walking.

In the standing position you want your structure to take most of the strai
your head should be looking straight ahead, so that there is minimal str?
It should feel like a gear stick in neutral. Shoulders should be neutr?
hunched forwards. Arms hanging loosely by the sides. Hips neutral. Legs unde₁ `.
slightly bent and over the toes. Toes should be pointing forwards.

drop the
you
n

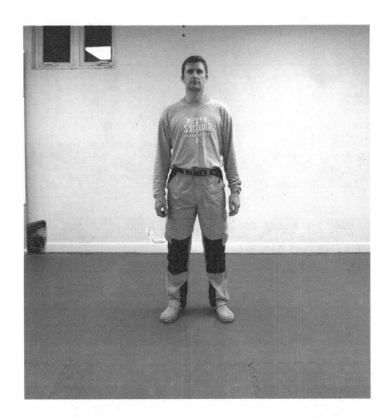

Just stand in this position, ideally in front of a mirror. Look at your posture in the mirror. It should be as even as possible (taking into consideration that no-one's posture is precisely even). If you draw a line down the middle of the body, both sides should be the same. Now close your eyes and try to feel any strain on muscles and relax this out with the breath.

You should now be standing with minimal effort to hold the posture.

Next you are going to understand more about your tension and how to release it. Often we are not aware that we are tense and the following exercise helps to highlight areas of tension and

...m out. Lean forwards slightly and notice where the tension picks up in the body to hold ...p. You will probably have already had some tension there. Pause, and then return to the ...utral position. As you return to the neutral position, notice the tension release. Often it is this tension release that really indicates where you are holding unnecessary tension.

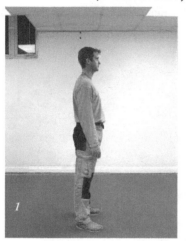 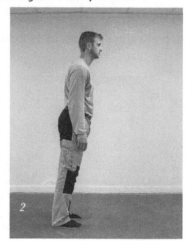

Do the same leaning backwards, side to side and the angles in between. Try to do all eight compass angles. Then move freely through all the angles, checking for and releasing tension.

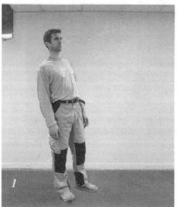 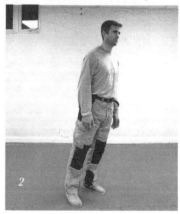

The Structure Walk

The good thing about this, is that you can practice this whenever you are walking, which should be a lot! When you walk in structure, there are five key things to think about.

1. **Breathing**: You can play with your breathing patterns from inhale one step, exhale one step to 2,3,4,5 6 or more. You can also do triangular and square breaths (see Practises 1 & 3). As before the aim is to stay as relaxed as possible during the inhale and relax all superfluous tension on the exhale. Practice a breath ladder up to 8 or 10, or as you improve 15 or 20 and then back down to 1 (See Practise 3).

2. **Take the body with you:** As you move practise keeping the chest above the feet. This is much better for balance and in a Martial Art it means that when you move, you take your whole body out of the danger area each time you move. As you move forwards, think about moving from the chest and as you move backwards, move from the chin.

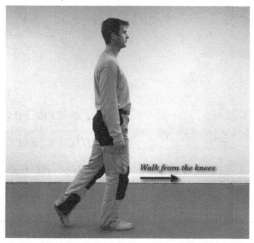

Walk from the knees

3. **Begin the step in the knees:** Think of the knees as the origin of the step. Bend the knees first and think about keeping the legs, especially the hips and feet, feeling light.

4. **Whole foot:** The whole foot lands at the same time. So you are not walking on the toes or the heels, but landing on your whole foot, so that you are completely centred and balanced in your walking.

5. **Relaxed:** Use the movement of walking to search for tension in your body and release it using the breath and light shrugging or wobbling movements. The aim is that each step makes you feel more relaxed.

To view the free video of this practise please use the link below:
http://www.matthill.co.uk/systema-health

"There are several ways to remove stress, the most important are breathing and movement."
- *Vladimir Vasiliev*

PRACTISE 17

SOFT FALLS

Do this once per day and you will not fear falling as you get older

As you go down to the floor try to make sure that you soften and relax the body as much as possible. You go down 'inside yourself' rather than spreading yourself out, so everything stays loose but compact.

Try to avoid pressure on your bones, such as hips, knees, elbows, ankles, and shoulders and keep the chin tucked in. As you go down, you 'collect' the body around a central point.

When you get to the ground you can extend the body out flat (this is only for training; in a real fall, there is obviously no need to do this, unless you are falling or rolling down a slope (for example skiing or scrambling) and you want to stop yourself. In this case you should make a star shape to get as much body contact as possible to stop yourself sliding.). Then collect the body around a point again and reverse the movement back to a standing position.

Important: Try to avoid pressure in the body, on your joints, tension in your muscles or holding your breath.

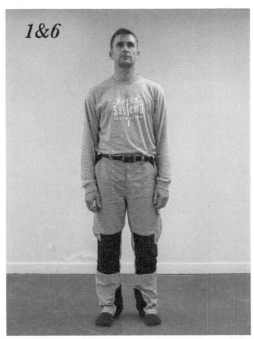

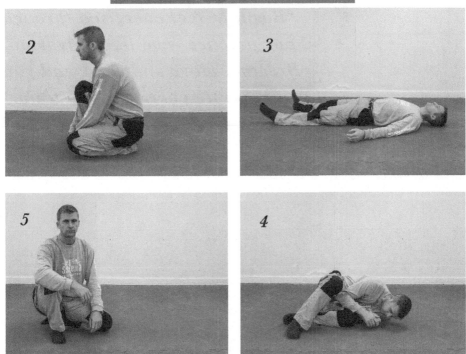

To view the free video of this practise please use the link below:

http://www.matthill.co.uk/systema-health

*"Begin to feel energised through
Your practice – be like a dynamo.
Breathe, move and relax and you
will generate energy as you train."*
                          -   Matt Hill

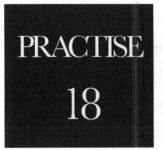

PRACTISE 18

ROLLING

Protection for the body

Rolling on the floor teaches you to protect your body as you fall. More than this, it gives you freedom of movement at ground level and is very healthy for the neck, shoulders, lower back and core.

Begin on the knees.

We begin on the knees, as this is less fearful for most people. Begin from instinct. If you fall forwards, your arms will naturally come out to protect you. We then turn this instinct into knowledge. Turn your head to the left side looking under your armpit.

FORWARDS ROLL

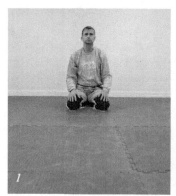
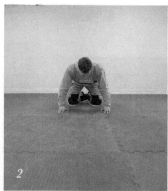
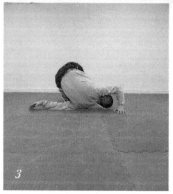

Rotate the right shoulder forwards and under you, by 'sweeping' the floor from inside to out and changing contact from the palm of the hand to the back of the hand. Use the toes of your right foot to push yourself over the top of your shoulders.

Your head should be tucked safely under your left arm. Now roll down the back and up to a sitting position.

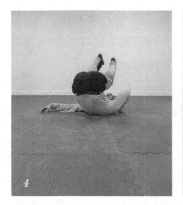

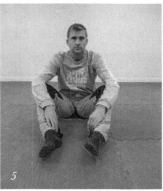

BACKWARDS ROLL

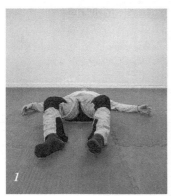

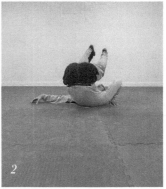

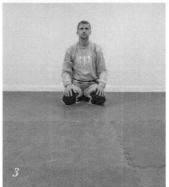

To do a backwards roll, you simply reverse the procedure as per the pictures. It is important that no pressure builds up on the head or neck. For this reason you roll over the shoulder, turning your head to look over the same shoulder at the last minute.

Once you get the hang of it, rolling on the floor is liberating. You can use it as a self-massage using the ground and gravity to ease out tension in your body.

Symmetry is important, so be sure to try rolling on your left and right sides.

Important. *As always it is very important that you exhale before you begin moving and keep the exhale going for the length of the roll. Inhale once you complete the roll and then exhale before you begin the backwards roll again, extending the breath for the length of the movement.*

To view the free video of this practise please use the link below:
http://www.matthill.co.uk/systema-health

PRACTISE

19

ROLLING FLAT

A challenging variation

A great variation on the rolling practise, is to move from your front to your back lengthways and vice versa. Begin by lying on your front, arms by your sides. Note that it is important that the head is turned so that the roll goes over the shoulder. Exhale and then begin to move from your core, with minimal effort and tension. Gradually draw your hips up over your head. Allow the legs to come all the way over the head and then slowly lower them using minimal tension and effort, until they are flat on the floor with you now lying on your back. Lead the movement with your breath on exhale. Then reverse the process to get back onto your front.

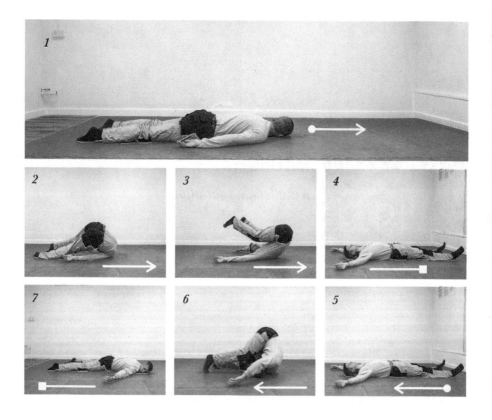

Note: This can be a good exercise to begin with, for those who are fearful of rolling, as the shoulder is already on the floor.

To view the free video of this practise please use the link below:

http://www.matthill.co.uk/systema-health

"The goal of training is not acquiring many quick and fancy moves, but learning to control your own pride irritation, fear, anger and self-pity."
- *Vladimir Vasiliev*

PRACTISE 20

ROLLING SIDEWAYS

Freedom and diversity in rolling

This movement practises you in the skill of rolling across the shoulders. It gives you the freedom to change direction in your rolls, bringing more diversity to the movement. It is also great for massaging the muscles of the upper back and neck. Begin sitting with your legs out straight. Exhale and fall to the side slowly. Reach out with your right hand, palm down. Rotate the arm palm up as your body comes to meet it, bringing the right knee towards the chest. Tuck the head under and continue the movement up onto the shoulders into the leg raise position. Come down onto the left side palm up, knee in and head on hand. Now rotate the arm back towards the ground palm down as you return to a sitting position. Try to exhale for the full extent of the movement.

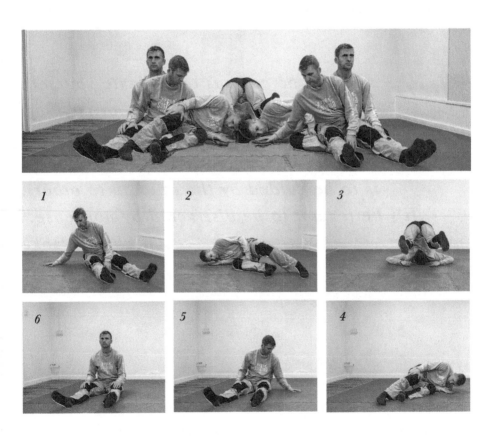

To view the free video of this practise please use the link below:
http://www.matthill.co.uk/systema-health

*"Always be curious to evaluate yourself,
your level of training.
Think about it.
Remember that the worst thing
is to be guided by the opinion to others.
It's better not to be distracted by nonsense."*
- Mikhail Ryabko

PRACTISE

21

BALANCE WALK

Progressing your relaxed walk

The balance walk practise is all about relaxation. For this practise, you simply walk forwards and backwards on a line. Walking forwards you walk heel to toe, left foot then right foot. Focus on your breathing and relaxing your muscles. Any tension will make you wobble and pull you off balance. Focus on maintaining full contact of your foot on the ground. Strive to keep your attention in the soles of the feet. To do this try to feel the ground through the soles of the feet in every step.

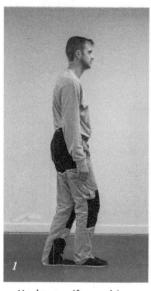 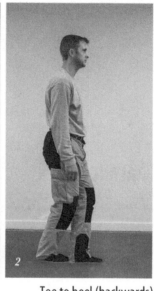 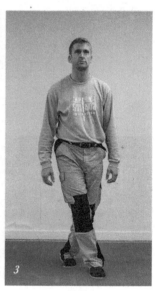

Heel to toe (forwards)   Toe to heel (backwards)   Crossing over

Next try walking backwards, toe to heel. When you can do it easily, try it with your eyes closed. Then try crossing the foot over the line each time with the same progressions. Further progressions can involve walking on a plank, tree branch or elevated beam.

To view the free video of this practise please use the link below:

http://www.matthill.co.uk/systema-health

"It is when you least want to get up and go train that you are going to get the most out of it personally."

- Matt Hill

PRACTISE

22

HEAVY DROPS

A surprisingly relaxing practise

The heavy drop practise helps you to learn to relax the body, especially the arms and legs. The aim is for the limbs to feel like a dead weight. This is a very good health and combat practise.

Begin lying on your back. Raise your arms up and hold them with minimal effort and tension. The shoulders should be relaxed and heavy against the floor. Exhale and drop the elbows, pause and then exhale and drop the hands. Do this several times. Then drop the whole arm at once.

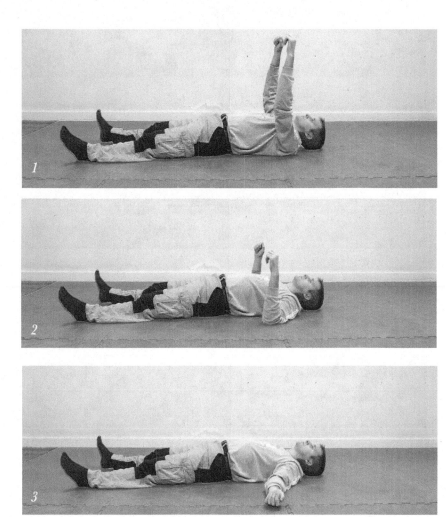

Now try it with the legs. Raise them to 90 degrees. First drop the heels to the bum, then extend the feet out straight to drop the legs. Be as heavy as possible in the legs.

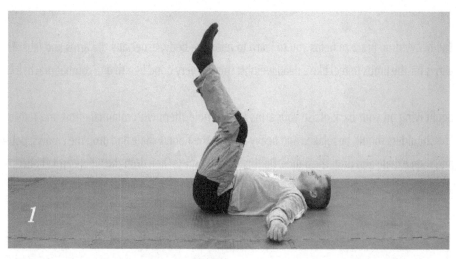

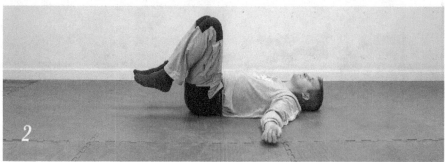

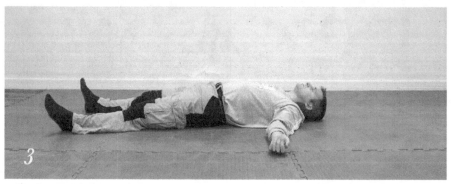

Again do this several times and then try the whole leg at once (be careful of your heels on hard floors).

Then try arms and legs at the same time. First elbows and heels, then hands and feet, then whole arm and leg at the same time.

The feel of the impact with the floor will highlight your areas of tension.

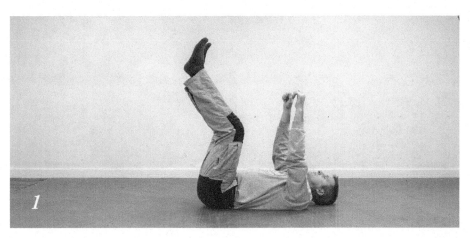

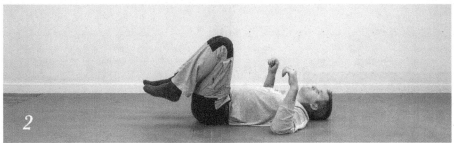

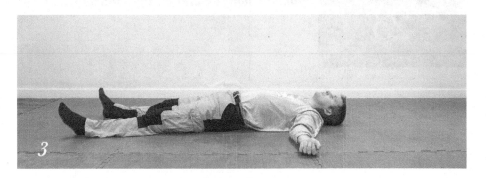

To view the free video of this practise please use the link below:

http://www.matthill.co.uk/systema-health

103

PRACTISE

23

ISOLATED TENSION

Building body awareness and control

The Isolated Tension practise builds body awareness and control. You will also become much more adept at finding and releasing tension from your body. Begin by lying on your back on the floor. This is a good position to start. You can of course do this standing, sitting or even walking. The best place for beginners however, is supine.

Inhale and tense the leg, from the toes to the gluteus muscles. Try to tense the whole leg at the same time. It is important that you isolate the tension in just that area. Hold the breath for a few seconds and then check the rest of the body for tension, using subtle movement or wobbling of the other muscles.

Next exhale and release the tension. Then try the right leg. Now try both legs at the same time. Then try the arm from the fingers to the shoulder. Then the other arm, then both arms at the same time. Again it is crucial that you isolate the tension, keeping the rest of the body relaxed.

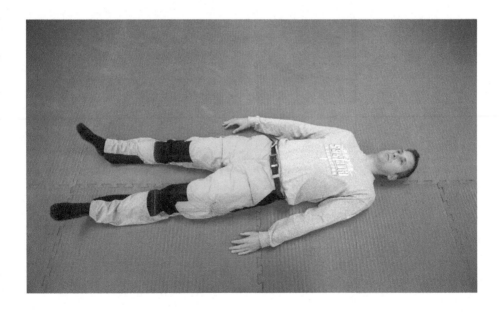

A big indicator is the exhale and release phase. Place your attention in the whole of the body as you relax. You will notice if other parts were tense, as you will feel them relax. Then try the stomach. Then the chest and back. Finally try the neck and head. Then try the whole of the top of the body from the waist up. Finally try the whole body.

When you can do this try to isolate the muscles even further. For example in the leg, try to tense just the foot.

Then do the same with the calf muscle. Systematically go all the way up the leg: knee, hamstring, quadriceps, glutes. Then try the whole leg in sequence, from the foot to the glutes.

You can also do a circuit from one foot to the other, sequentially tensing the muscles and then releasing them in reverse. Also do this with the arms (hands, forearms, elbow, bicep, tricep and shoulder) and torso (stomach, chest, latissimus, lower back, upper back) neck and head. This is difficult and takes some practise.

To view the free video of this practise please use the link below:
http://www.matthill.co.uk/systema-health

*"Tension in your body
is a manifestation of
fear at some level."*
- Mikhail Ryabko

PRACTISE

24

TENSION WAVE

Learning to feel tension build and then learning to let it drain away

This is similar to the last practise, but this time you imagine your body as a vessel filling up with tension and then draining of tension. Begin in the toes and on one inhale, gradually fill the body with tension from bottom to top.

Hold and feel full tension in the body, then release the tension back towards the feet. Try it in reverse from head to toe, from right fingers to left fingers and left fingers to right fingers.

Another way to imagine it is like an MRI, scan where the red line fills you with tension as it passes from the head to the toes and then vice versa.

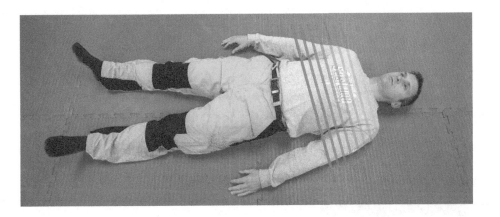

To view the free video of this practise please use the link below:
http://www.matthill.co.uk/systema-health

PRACTISE

25

TENSION LESSENING

Understanding how tension builds, and how to 'head it off at the pass'

The final practise is one of the most beneficial, as it shows you how to relax deeply. You go will go beneath muscle tension and get to the root cause of tension, the nervous system. Begin the practise by lying on your back.

Over an inhale of three-seconds, gradually bring 100% tension to every muscle in the body. As tense as you possibly can. Hold for three-seconds then exhale for three-seconds.

Important note: *this can also be done for other counts e.g. 1, 5, 8, 10 etc., or in an instant such as a clap.*

Now do the same exercise for 90% tension, then 80%, then 70% etc. If you are short of time you can do (80, 60, 40 etc.) Go all the way to 10%. Really try to think about what 80%, 50% 30% etc., mean. At 10% the muscles barely engage in tension. Then try to do 1% tension. No muscles should engage at this point.

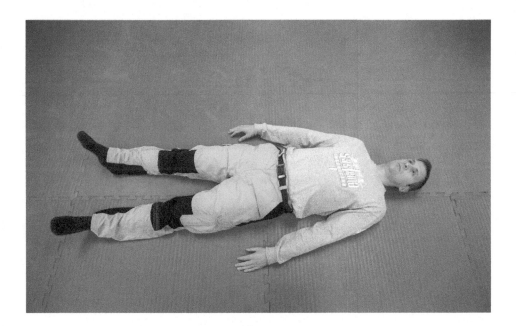

At 1% you just send the signal to them to tense. The body should feel like a current is going around it, but it does not engage any muscles. Hold this for the count of three, then release. If you feel a release at this point, that is your nervous system. When you can learn to feel this begin to engage, and then consciously release it, you are starting to feel the root cause of tension. When you understand this, you can start to stop tension before it becomes a problem. You can 'head it off at the pass.'

To view the free video of this practise please use the link below:

http://www.matthill.co.uk/systema-health

IN CONCLUSION
Progression on your journey

It is my hope that you will continue your exploration through the concepts outlined in this book over the coming months and years. This book is just a catalyst for further research and practice. As Bruce Lee famously said, 'Use only that which works and take it from any place you can find it.'

The drills outlined in the pages of this book are not meant to be dogmatic. Systema is not a 'frozen' Martial Art. It is continually evolving. With each new person that comes to it, it evolves again. These drills can and should be adapted and mixed with your own experience and knowledge. The permutations are limitless.

If you wish to progress further in your journey you should seek out a good instructor. Vladimir Vasiliev has a useful instructor search tool on his website:

https://www.russianmartialart.com/schoollocator.php

Try not to get frustrated in your progress. I wish you fortune, strength, health and happiness in your journey.

If you have any questions please feel free to contact me through the website www.matthill.co.uk or email wiltshiremartialarts@gmail.com.

Don't forget to get access to your complimentary video of each of the practises outlined in the book by using this link: http://www.matthill.co.uk/systema-health

Recommended Reading:

Let Every Breath - Vladimir Vasiliev.
Strikes, Soul Meets Body - Vladimir Vasiliev.

Recommended Viewing:

Both Mikhail Ryabko and Vladimir Vasiliev have extensive video collections. Videos for both teachers can be found and purchased from their websites.

Notes

Notes

Notes

Notes

Made in the USA
Las Vegas, NV
17 February 2023

67701958R00069